YOGA FOR WOMEN OVER 40

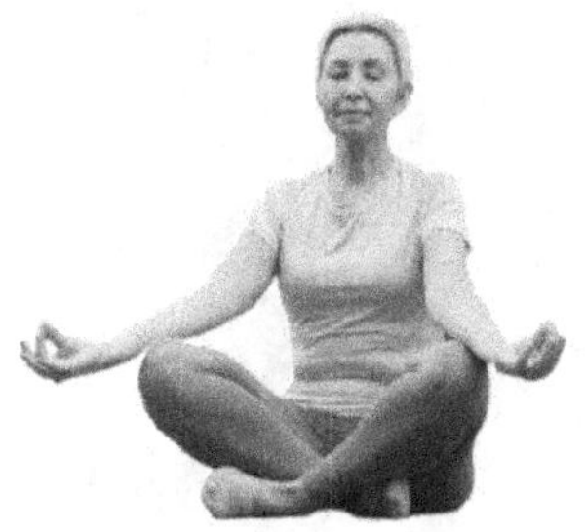

Dr. Mary Dixon

Copyright © 2023 by Dr. Mary Dixon

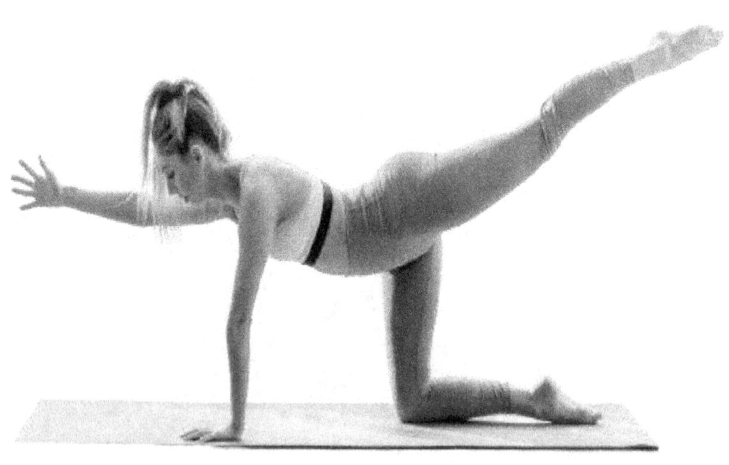

Table of Contents

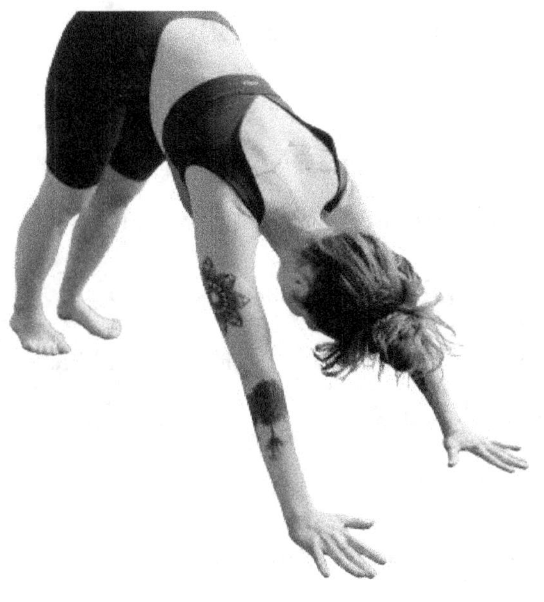

INTRODUCTION

There was a woman named Sarah who had a history of fitness issues. She had tried various exercises and diets over the years, but nothing seemed to work for her. One day, a buddy advised her to give yoga a try.

At first, Sarah was sceptical. She had always thought of yoga as something only hippies did. But her friend was insistent, and eventually, Sarah agreed to give it a try.

To her surprise, Sarah found that she really enjoyed yoga. It was both demanding and calming at the same time. She loved the way it made her feel both physically and mentally.

As she continued to practice, Sarah started to notice changes in her body. She felt stronger and more flexible, and she had more energy throughout the day. She also found that she was more focused and less stressed.

Sarah started going to yoga classes regularly, and she even started doing some yoga at home on her own. Over time, she became more and more skilled, and she was able to do poses that she never thought possible.

But the real payoff came when Sarah went on a hiking trip with some friends. In the past, Sarah had always struggled to keep up with the group, but this time was different. Thanks to her newfound fitness and stamina from yoga, Sarah was able to hike for hours without feeling tired or out of breath.

As Sarah stood at the top of a mountain, taking in the breathtaking view, she realized that yoga had truly changed her life. She felt stronger, healthier, and happier than ever before, and she knew that she would continue practicing yoga for years to come.

Yoga is a traditional exercise that has been practiced for thousands of years and has its roots in India. It is a holistic approach to health and well-being that combines physical postures, breath control, meditation, and ethical principles. The word yoga means "union" in Sanskrit, and it is often described as a union of the mind, body, and spirit.

The practice of yoga has gained popularity in recent years, as people have discovered its numerous benefits for physical, mental, and emotional health. Yoga can be practiced by people of all ages and fitness levels, and it can be adapted to suit individual needs and abilities.

Yoga can increase strength and flexibility, which is one of its key advantages. The physical postures, or asanas, are designed to stretch and strengthen the muscles, joints, and ligaments of the body. This can help to reduce pain and stiffness, improve range of motion, and prevent injury.

Another effective method for lowering stress and anxiety is yoga. The deep breathing techniques and meditation practices can help to calm the mind and promote relaxation. This can lead to a greater sense of well-being and improved mental clarity.

In addition to its physical and mental benefits, yoga also promotes a sense of connection and community. Many people find that practicing yoga in a group setting can be a great way to meet new people and build relationships.

Overall, yoga is a powerful tool for improving health and well-being. Whether you are looking to improve your flexibility, reduce stress, or simply connect with others, yoga can be a great addition to your wellness routine.

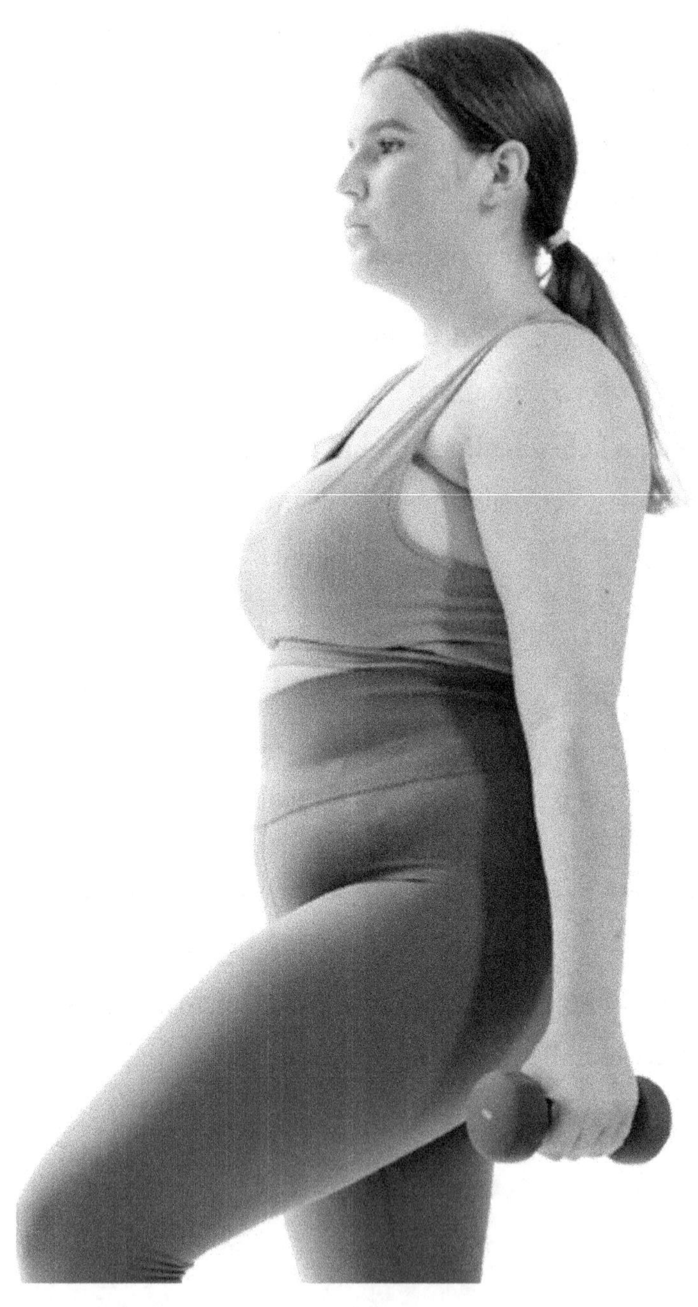

CHAPTER ONE

Benefits of Yoga for Women Over 40

Yoga is a great way for women over 40 to stay active and maintain good health. It is a form of exercise that promotes physical and mental wellbeing, and can provide a number of benefits for women who are entering middle age. Here are some of the key benefits of yoga for women over 40:

Increased flexibility and mobility

As we age, our joints tend to become stiffer, and we may experience a loss of flexibility and mobility. Yoga can help to counteract these effects by stretching and strengthening the muscles and joints. This can lead to greater ease of movement and improved posture.

Reduced stress and anxiety

Middle age can be a stressful time, with many women facing a range of challenges such as caring for aging parents, navigating career changes, and dealing with hormonal changes. Yoga can provide a calming and grounding effect, helping to reduce stress and anxiety. Regular yoga practice has been shown to lower levels of the stress hormone cortisol, and can also improve sleep quality.

Improved bone density

As women age, they are at increased risk of developing osteoporosis, a condition in which bones become brittle and fragile. Weight-bearing exercises like yoga can help to maintain or improve bone density, reducing the risk of fractures and falls.

Better balance and coordination

Yoga poses require balance and coordination, which can help to improve these skills as we age. This can be particularly important for women over 40, as falls become more common with age. Improved balance and coordination can reduce the risk of falls and injuries.

Reduced inflammation

Heart disease, diabetes, and cancer are just a few of the health issues that chronic inflammation has been associated to. Regular yoga practice has been shown to reduce inflammation in the body, which can have a range of positive health benefits.

Improved cardiovascular health

Yoga can provide a gentle cardiovascular workout, helping to improve heart health and reduce the risk of heart disease. Some styles of yoga, such as vinyasa or power yoga, can be particularly beneficial for cardiovascular health.

Increased mindfulness and self-awareness

Yoga is often described as a practice that promotes mindfulness and self-awareness. By tuning in to the breath and the body, women over 40 can develop greater awareness of their physical and emotional states. This can help to improve overall wellbeing and lead to greater self-acceptance and self-compassion.

Reduced menopausal symptoms

Many women experience a range of symptoms during menopause, such as hot flashes, mood swings, and insomnia. Yoga has been shown to reduce the severity and frequency of these symptoms, helping women to manage the transition more smoothly.

Improved digestion

Yoga poses and breathing techniques can help to stimulate the digestive system, improving digestion and reducing symptoms such as bloating and constipation.

Greater sense of community

Yoga classes can provide a supportive community of like-minded individuals, which can be particularly important for women over 40 who may be experiencing a sense of isolation or loneliness. The sense of connection and belonging that comes from practicing yoga with others can be incredibly beneficial for overall wellbeing.

In conclusion, yoga can provide a range of benefits for women over 40, from increased flexibility and mobility to reduced stress and improved cardiovascular health.

Whether practiced at home or in a studio setting, yoga can be a valuable tool for maintaining good health and wellbeing throughout middle age and beyond.

CHAPTER TWO

Yoga Positions for Women Over 40

Mountain Pose (Tad asana)

With your arms at your sides and your palms facing forward, take a tall stance.

Tree Pose (Vrksasana)

Stand with your feet hip-width apart, shift your weight to your left foot, place your right foot on your left thigh, and balance.

Warrior I (Virabhadrasana I)

Stand with your feet hip-width apart, step your left foot back, bend your right knee, and raise your arms overhead.

Warrior II (Virabhadrasana II)

From Warrior I, open your hips to the side, extend your arms out to the sides, and gaze over your front hand.

Triangle Pose (Trikonasana)

Stand with your feet wide apart, extend your arms out to the sides, and reach your right hand towards your right foot.

Half Moon Pose (Ardha Chandrasana)

From Triangle Pose, place your left hand on your left hip, lift your right leg, and reach your right hand towards the ceiling.

Downward-Facing Dog Pose (Adho Mukha Svanasana)

Start on your hands and knees, curl your toes under, lift your hips, and extend your arms and legs.

Child's Pose (Balasana)

From Downward-Facing Dog, drop your knees to the mat, sit back on your heels, and extend your arms forward.

Cobra Pose (Bhujangasana)

Lie on your stomach, place your hands under your shoulders, and lift your chest off the mat.

Upward-Facing Dog Pose (Urdhva Mukha Svanasana)

From Cobra Pose, straighten your arms, lift your hips off the mat, and roll over your toes.

Camel Pose (Ustrasana)

Kneel on the mat, place your hands on your lower back, and arch your back as you lift your chest and gaze towards the ceiling.

Pigeon Pose (Eka Pada Rajakapotasana)

Start on your hands and knees, bring your right knee behind your right wrist, and extend your left leg behind you.

Seated Forward Bend (Paschimottanasana)

Sit on the mat with your legs extended in front of you, fold forward from your hips, and reach for your toes.

Wide-Legged Forward Bend (Prasarita Padottanasana)

Stand with your feet wide apart, fold forward from your hips, and place your hands on the mat.

Lord of the Fishes Half Pose (Ardha Matsyendrasana)

Sit on the mat with your legs extended in front of you, bend your right knee, place your right foot on the mat, and twist to the right.

Bridge Pose (Setu Bandhasana)

Lie on your back, bend your knees, place your feet on the mat, and lift your hips.

Fish Pose (Matsyasana)

Lie on your back, place your hands under your hips, arch your back, and lift your chest towards the ceiling.

Corpse Pose (Savasana)

Lie on your back with your legs extended and arms at your sides, close your eyes, and relax your entire body.

Eagle Pose (Garudasana)

Stand tall, lift your right leg, cross your right thigh over your left thigh, and wrap your right foot around your left calf. Then, bring your hands together, bend your elbows, and cross your right arm over your left.

Cow Face Pose (Gomukhasana)

Sit on the mat with your legs extended in front of you, bend your right knee, and place your right foot on the mat next to your left hip. Then, bend your left knee, cross your left leg over your right leg, and place your left foot on the mat next to your right hip. Your right arm should be extended upwards toward the sky. Bend your elbow and place your hand behind your back. Then, reach your left arm behind your back, bend your elbow, and bring your hand up towards your right hand. Clasp your hands together, if possible.

Camel Pose with a Block (Ustrasana)

Kneel on the mat with a block behind you, place your hands on your lower back, and arch your back as you lift your chest and gaze towards the ceiling. Place your hands on the block for support.

Chair Pose (Utkatasana)

Stand tall, raise your arms overhead, and bend your knees as if you are sitting in a chair.

Revolved Triangle Pose (Parivrtta Trikonasana)

Stand with your feet hip-width apart, extend your arms out to the sides, and reach your right hand towards your left foot. Twist your torso to the left and gaze towards your left hand.

Extended Triangle Pose (Utthita Trikonasana)

Stand with your feet wide apart, extend your arms out to the sides, and reach your right hand towards your right foot. Gaze towards your left hand.

Extended Side Angle Pose (Utthita Parsvakonasana)

From Warrior II, place your right hand on the mat next to your right foot and reach your left arm towards the ceiling.

Garland Pose (Malasana)

Squat on the mat with your feet together and your heels on the mat. Put your hands at your heart in a position of prayer.

Goddess Pose (Utkata Konasana)

Stand with your feet wide apart, turn your toes out, and bend your knees. Place your hands on your hips or raise your arms overhead.

Reclining Bound Angle Pose (Supta Baddha Konasana)

Kneel down on the floor with your feet together and your soles touching. Your knees should be free to fall open to the sides.

Head-to-Knee Forward Bend (Janu Sirsasana)

Sit on the mat with your left leg extended in front of you and your right knee bent. Put your right foot's sole up against your left thigh. Fold forward from your hips and reach for your left foot.

Wide-Angle Seated Forward Bend (Upavistha Konasana)

Sit on the mat with your legs extended wide apart. Fold forward from your hips and reach for your toes.

Shoulder Stand (Sarvangasana)

Lie on your back, lift your legs overhead, and support your back with your hands.

Plow Pose (Halasana)

From Shoulder Stand, lower your legs behind your head and place your feet on the mat.

Fish Pose with a Block (Matsyasana)

Lie on your back with a block under your shoulder blades. Arch your back, lift your chest towards the ceiling, and relax Supported Bridge Pose (Setu Bandha Sarvangasana)

Knees bowed and feet flat on the mat, lie on your back. Lift your hips towards the ceiling and place a block under your sacrum.

Half Frog Pose (Ardha Bhekasana)

Lie on your stomach, bend your right knee, and reach back with your right hand to grab your right foot. Press your foot into your hand and lift your knee off the mat.

Pigeon Pose (Eka Pada Rajakapotasana)

Start on your hands and knees, bring your right knee forward and place it behind your right wrist. Straighten your left leg behind you and lower your torso onto your front leg.

Butterfly Pose (Baddha Konasana)

Sit on the mat with the soles of your feet together and knees bent out to the sides. Bring your heels as close to your body as possible and fold forward from your hips.

Revolved Head-to-Knee Pose (Parivrtta Janu Sirsasana)

Sit with your left leg extended and right knee bent. Place your right foot against your left inner thigh. Reach your left hand toward your right foot while rotating your torso to the right.

Seated Forward Bend (Paschimottanasana)

Sit on the mat with your legs extended in front of you. Fold forward from your hips and reach for your feet.

Legs-Up-the-Wall Pose (Viparita Karani)

Your legs should be extended up the wall while you lay on your back.

Easy Pose with Forward Fold (Sukhasana with Paschimottanasana)

Sit on the mat with your legs crossed and fold forward from your hips.

Gate Pose (Parighasana)

Kneel on the mat with your left knee forward and right leg extended to the side. Reach your right arm up towards the ceiling and bend to the left.

Side Plank Pose (Vasisthasana)

Start in a plank pose, shift your weight onto your left hand and outer edge of your left foot. Stack your right foot on top of your left foot and reach your right arm towards the ceiling.

Bow Pose (Dhanurasana)

Lie on your stomach, bend your knees, and reach back to grab your ankles. Off the mat, raise your thighs and chest.

Upward Facing Dog Pose (Urdhva Mukha Svanasana)

Lie on your stomach with your hands under your shoulders, press into your hands and lift your chest and thighs off the mat.

Downward Facing Dog Pose (Adho Mukha Svanasana)

Begin by getting down on all fours, tucking your toes, and lifting your hips upward.

Extended Puppy Pose (Uttana Shishosana)

Start in a tabletop position, walk your hands forward and lower your chest towards the mat.

Extended Hand-to-Big-Toe Pose (Utthita Hasta Padangustasana)

Stand with your feet hip-width apart, lift your right leg and hold onto your big toe with your right hand. Extend your right leg in front of you.

Pyramid Pose (Parsvottanasana)

Stand with your feet hip-width apart, step your left foot back, and fold forward over your right leg.

Warrior III Pose (Virabhadrasana III)

Stand with your feet hip-width apart, lift your left leg behind you, and hinge forward from your hips. Reach your arms forward.

CONCLUSION

In conclusion, yoga is an excellent practice for women over 40 due to its numerous physical, mental, and emotional benefits. As women age, their bodies undergo various changes that can affect their overall health and well-being. Yoga can help alleviate some of these changes and improve overall health and fitness.

Through regular practice of yoga, women over 40 can improve their flexibility, balance, and strength, which can help reduce the risk of falls and injuries. It can also help relieve joint pain, stiffness, and other age-related health issues such as arthritis. Additionally, yoga can help reduce stress levels and improve sleep quality, which is essential for maintaining overall health.

Yoga also provides women with an opportunity to connect with themselves on a deeper level. As women age, they may experience changes in their relationships, career, and personal goals.

Yoga can provide a sense of inner peace and calmness that can help them navigate these changes with greater ease.

Furthermore, yoga can help women over 40 develop a greater sense of body awareness and acceptance. This can be particularly helpful for women who may have struggled with body image issues throughout their lives. Through yoga, women can learn to appreciate their bodies for what they are and become more comfortable in their own skin.

Finally, yoga is a highly accessible practice that can be done virtually anywhere, making it ideal for women over 40 who may have busy schedules or mobility issues.

With the availability of online yoga classes, women can practice at home or while traveling, making it easier to incorporate into their daily lives.

Overall, yoga is a highly beneficial practice for women over 40. Whether they are looking to improve their physical health, reduce stress, or connect with themselves on a deeper level, yoga can provide numerous benefits that can help them feel their best at any age.

With its accessibility, flexibility, and adaptability, yoga is an ideal practice for women looking to maintain and improve their health and well-being well into their golden years.

www.ingramcontent.com/pod-product-compliance
Lightning Source LLC
Chambersburg PA
CBHW060910260726
48661CB00008B/3568